CANCER AND MODERN SCIENCE™

SKIN CANCER

Current and Emerging Trends in Detection and Treatment

TRACIE EGAN

The Rosen Publishing Group, Inc., New York

Published in 2006 by The Rosen Publishing Group, Inc.
29 East 21st Street, New York, NY 10010

First Edition

Library of Congress Cataloging-in-Publication Data

Egan, Tracie.
Skin cancer: current and emerging trends in detection and treatment/
by Tracie Egan.—1st ed.
    p. cm.—(Cancer and modern science)
Includes bibliographical references and index.
ISBN 1-4042-0390-7 (library binding)
1. Melanoma—Juvenile literature.
I. Title. II. Series.
RC280.M37E36 2006
616.99'477—dc22

                                                                2004025553

Manufactured in Malaysia

On the cover: Colored scanning electron micrograph (SEM) of skin cancer cells.

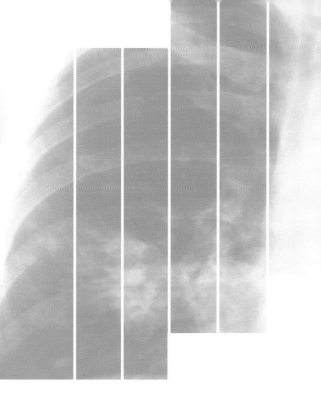
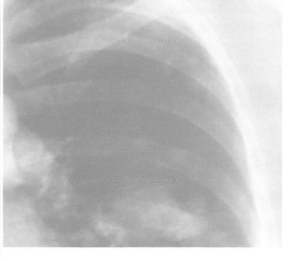

CONTENTS

INTRODUCTION

Skin cancer is exactly what its name suggests: cancer that initiates in the skin. It is the most common form of cancer in the United States, which isn't that surprising, considering that the skin is the largest organ of the human body. Of the three main types of skin cancer—basal cell carcinoma, squamous cell carcinoma, and malignant melanoma (referred to simply as melanoma)—malignant melanoma is the most dangerous. Like basal cell and squamous cell carcinoma (both of which are referred to as nonmelanoma), melanoma generally begins on sun-exposed surfaces of the skin, but unlike nonmelanoma, it has the ability to spread very quickly to other parts of the body.

Skin cancer is diagnosed through the detection of lesions on the surface of the skin. Melanoma lesions usually start off as pigmented moles on the skin that, over time, begin to change in size, shape, or color; become itchy; or begin to bleed. The number of people diagnosed with skin cancer rises each year, but the disease has a very low fatality rate. While nonmelanoma is the most common form of skin cancer,

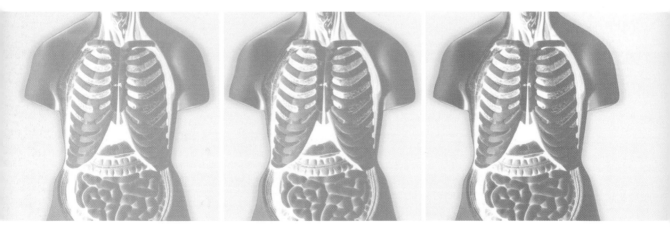

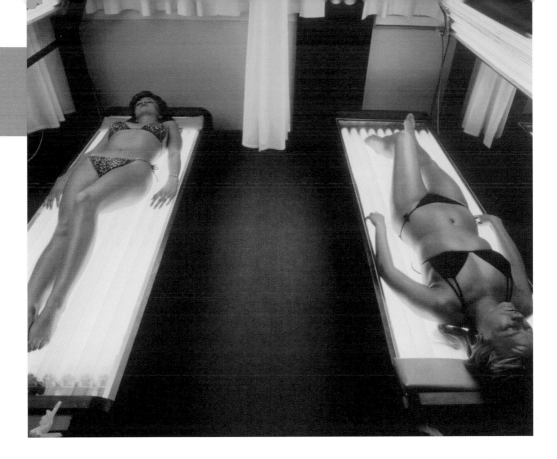

Exposure to the sun increases the risk of skin cancer. Although some people think tanning in booths is a way around that, the truth is that tanning booths deliver ultraviolet rays that can be just as dangerous as spending time in the sun. The best way to avoid skin cancer is to limit exposure altogether.

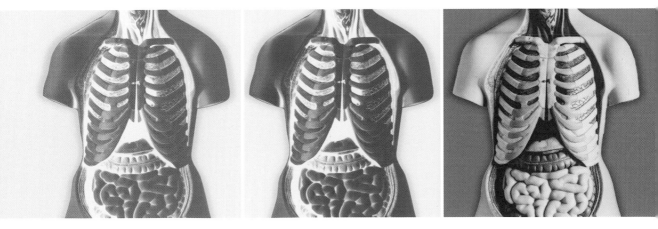

melanoma is responsible for most skin cancer–related deaths. Fortunately, due to medical research and advances, melanoma is preventable and treatable. Taking an active role—such as monitoring sun exposure and periodically examining moles on your body—could make all the difference. The key to successful prevention and treatment is understanding how to protect your skin from damage, and knowing what to look for in order to detect the disease at an early stage.

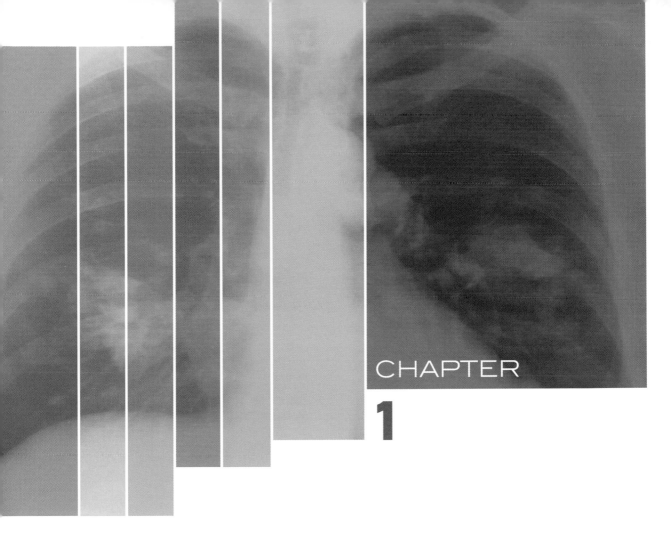

THE BASICS OF SKIN CANCER

The skin is actually an organ—the largest in the body—and it does more than just help keep your blood and bones inside of you. Skin helps protect us from our environment, helps regulate our body temperature, and is able to sense touch, temperature, and pain. Your hair and nails are also a part of your skin. The skin is made up of two layers: the epidermis (the outer layer), primarily made up of basal and squamous cells, and the dermis, which is made up of connective tissue and lies beneath the epidermis.

THE EPIDERMIS AND THE DERMIS

Normal, everyday activity can cause stress to the skin. In order to deal with this stress, your body must replace skin cells each day. This is the job of basal cells. Basal cells are long and thin and are found in the lowest layer of the epidermis. As basal cells reproduce, there is not enough room for the new cells, so some of the cells are pushed toward the top of the epidermis. As they move upward, the basal cells flatten and turn into squamous cells. Squamous cells are packed close together and, depending on the area, form a thick layer called the cornified layer. Located in the lowest level of the epidermis with basal cells are melanocytes, cells that make melanin. Melanin is the pigment that determines the color of your skin. Melanin is able to absorb ultraviolet (UV) rays from the sun, which changes the pigment of your skin. Most melanocytes are found in the skin, but they can also be found in the brain, eyes, or lining of the mouth, vagina, and rectum.

Below the epidermis is the dermis, which is mostly made up of connective tissue that is divided into two layers: papillary tissue and reticular tissue. The dermis is full of blood and lymphatic vessels. (The lymphatic system produces disease-fighting cells known as lymphocytes for the immune system.) Below the dermis is subcutaneous tissue that contains organs such as glands for sweating, hair follicles, blood and lymphatic vessels, and nerves.

THE SCIENCE OF CANCER

All types of cancer are rooted in the principle that mutations in DNA cause uncontrolled cell growth. The smallest form of life is the cell. All living things, from trees to fungi and dogs to humans, are composed of cells. Humans are made up of millions of cells. Cells reproduce by splitting and forming new cells. Inside every cell is material known as deoxyribonucleic acid, or DNA. DNA creates a code that determines everything that

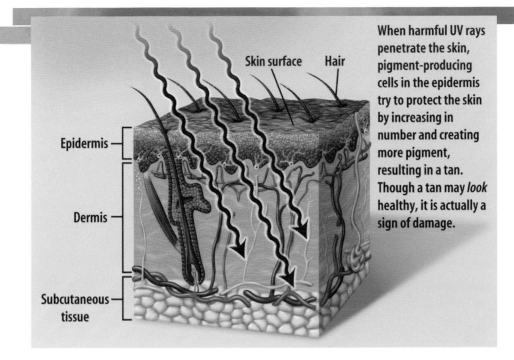

Skin surface Hair

Epidermis

Dermis

Subcutaneous tissue

When harmful UV rays penetrate the skin, pigment-producing cells in the epidermis try to protect the skin by increasing in number and creating more pigment, resulting in a tan. Though a tan may *look* healthy, it is actually a sign of damage.

This illustration shows the three main layers of the skin: the epidermis, dermis, and subcutaneous tissue. When UV rays from the sun are absorbed into the epidermis, the cells there produce more pigment, resulting in tanned skin.

happens within the cell. This code is organized in your genes. Units of DNA known as genes are passed on to you from your parents and are responsible for certain traits, such as your appearance.

Cancer is a condition in which a body uncontrollably reproduces a particular kind of cell, even when there is no need for additional cells. This uncontrollable reproduction is caused by errors in the DNA. There are two ways this can happen. The first is a mistake in copying DNA during cell division. This type of error is inherited from your parents. The second is when DNA becomes damaged from an external source—either chemical or physical—and is incorrectly repaired by enzymes. Mistakes made in duplicating DNA are known as mutations.

As basal cells in the epidermis are being lost and replaced, a genetic mutation can cause the new cells to be cancerous. These mutations that make a person more susceptible to skin cancer can be inherited from your parents. More often, they can be caused by damage to the DNA code by an external source, namely ultraviolet rays from the sun.

THE THREE TYPES OF SKIN CANCER

As mentioned earlier, there are three main types of skin cancer: basal cell carcinoma, squamous cell carcinoma, and malignant melanoma. Over 80 percent of skin cancer cases are due to basal cell carcinoma. Though it is the most common form of skin cancer in the United States, it is extremely rare for basal cell carcinoma to result in death. A basal cell carcinoma is pearl colored and raised with visible blood vessels within the lesion. Skin surfaces that are exposed to the sun are more susceptible to

THE HISTORY OF MELANOMA

Melanoma has been recognized as a disease for as far back as 400 BC. Hippocrates (460–377 BC), the Greek physician regarded as the father of medicine, referred to it as a black tumor. Melanoma was first documented and treated, albeit unsuccessfully, in Western medicine by British physician John Hunter in 1787. It wasn't until 1905, that Samson Handley, a research fellow at a London hospital, made the first real advance in the treatment of malignant melanoma. Applying his research of metastasized breast cancer to melanoma, Handley removed the tumor and the subcutaneous tissue surrounding it, setting the standard for surgical management of melanoma for years to come.

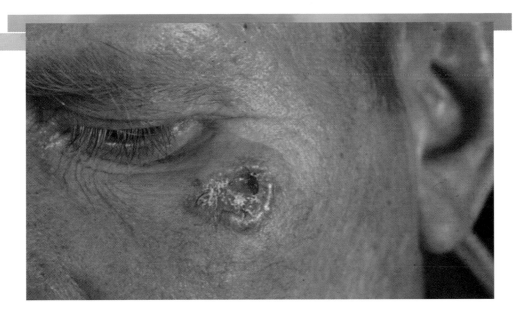

This man has a basal cell carcinoma on his cheek. Basal cell carcinomas are the most common and the least threatening types of skin cancer. Note that the basal cell carcinomas are most often found on the face and are easy to see with the naked eye.

basal cell carcinomas, but they occur mostly on the face. The lesion invades locally at a very slow rate, but if left untreated, the lesions can be extremely destructive to the skin.

Squamous cell carcinoma is the second most common form of skin cancer, and, if detected early, is curable in almost all cases. But if left untreated, it is capable of spreading locally, and it can be deadly. A squamous cell carcinoma typically starts off hard, crusty, and scaly, and normally has an ulcer in the center, with raised, red borders surrounding the ulcer. Like basal cell carcinomas, squamous cell carcinomas are most common on sun-exposed surfaces of the skin.

Malignant melanoma attacks the body differently from basal and squamous cell carcinomas. When a cancer is malignant, it means that it

Normal Mole	Melanoma	Sign	Characteristic
		Asymmetry	When half of the mole does not match the other half
		Border	When the border (edges) of the mole are ragged or irregular
		Color	When the color of the mole varies throughout
		Diameter	If the mole's diameter is larger than a pencil's eraser

Doctors have devised a system that describes characteristics of melanomas. Called the ABCD (or ABCDE) Chart, the photographs above clearly show the difference between healthy moles and melanomas that may be asymmetrical, have an irregular border, have differences in color, or have a large diameter. This system is further explained in chapter 4.

is life threatening. While basal and squamous cell cancers tend to invade locally and remain at the point of invasion, melanoma spreads quickly to other parts of the body. This process of a cancer cell leaving the area where it began and moving to other parts of the body is known as metastasis. Although melanoma does not start off as malignant, once it has progressed to a certain phase, it will spread and become malignant. It is the ability to metastasize that separates melanoma from non-melanoma skin cancer.

Melanoma is cancer of the melanocytes, the cells that make melanin, and is the deadliest form of skin cancer. Like nonmelanoma, melanoma typically affects sun-exposed areas of the skin. Yet, in rare cases, it can occur on mucous surfaces, like the mouth, vagina, or rectum.

Melanoma lesions are normally pigmented in shades of brown or black, appearing to be moles. However, in about 10 percent of melanoma cases, patients have amelanotic lesions. An amelanotic lesion is a melanoma that doesn't make pigment, and thus, is flesh colored.

RISK FACTORS

Factors such as genetics, gender, race, age, and geographic location can contribute to whether or not a person is likely to develop skin cancer. Melanoma is most common in people older than forty, with chances increasing as an individual gets older. It almost exclusively affects light-skinned Caucasians over people of races with darker complexions. While these factors all contribute to the risk for melanoma, what really causes a person to develop skin cancer is damage caused by UV rays from the sun. The ozone layer is our first defense against UV rays. However, the depletion of the

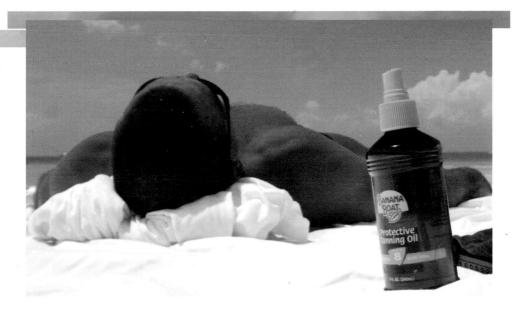

Even though exposure to the sun is well known to be the greatest risk for developing skin cancer, it is unrealistic to think that people will stay inside all day. However, limiting exposure to the sun should be considered, and protecting oneself from harmful rays should become a daily habit. Aside from hats and clothing, one good way to protect skin is to use sunscreen and sunblock.

ozone layer due to pollution has increased our exposure to UV rays, resulting in more cases of skin cancer each year.

The increased exposure to UV rays, coupled with fashion trends such as skin tanning and clothing that reveals more skin, has made melanoma the fastest rising cancer in the United States. The percentage of people who develop melanoma has more than doubled in the past thirty years. Each year, more than 50,000 cases are diagnosed. According to the Melanoma Research Foundation, one out of seventy-five Americans will develop melanoma at some point in their lives. In the United States, one person dies every hour from melanoma, according to a 1996 report released by the American Academy of Dermatology (AAD).

BIOLOGICAL RISK FACTORS

There are six different skin types, based on color and likelihood of tanning and burning. Skin type is determined at birth and is set for life. Four of the six types are more likely to develop skin cancer or melanoma. Type 1 is white skin that always burns, freckles easily, and is the most likely to develop melanoma. Type 2 is white skin that usually burns and freckles, and tans with difficulty. Type 2 is the second most likely skin type to develop melanoma. Type 3 is white skin that sometimes burns but mostly tans. Type 3 is less vulnerable to melanoma than Type 1 or 2. Type 4, usually belonging to people of Mediterranean descent, is white skin that tans easily and never burns, and is not very likely to develop melanoma. A general rule of thumb is that the darker the skin color, the lower the risk of developing skin cancer. However, it's important to remember that low risk does not mean no risk.

While people with a family history of melanoma are at a high risk for developing the disease themselves, melanoma itself can't be passed down from one family member to another. However, the risks of developing melanoma can be inherited through certain types of genes, like skin type, eye color, and hair color. For instance, people with red hair are twice as likely to develop melanoma than those with dark hair. A common inherited risk factor is the dysplastic nevus syndrome (also known as familial atypical mole melanoma syndrome). Dysplastic moles are abnormal moles in that they are larger than normal moles, with irregular shapes and multiple colors. These moles are hereditary. Sometimes dysplastic moles develop into a malignancy, but in most cases, dysplastic moles serve as an indicator in identifying those who have an increased risk of a melanoma somewhere else on their body. In other words, a person who has a dysplastic mole on his or her body is at a higher risk for developing melanoma than a person who does not have a dysplastic mole.

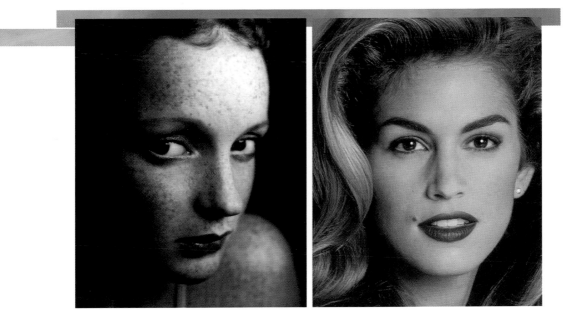

Some people are more likely to develop skin cancer than others, and those people should be even more careful to protect themselves from harmful UV rays. Fair-skinned Caucasians are most at risk, especially those who are freckled like the girl on the left. Famous model Cindy Crawford's (right) mole helped her make millions, but such moles can turn malignant and should be regularly checked.

When a child is born with a mole, it is called a congenital mole. Congenital moles don't necessarily indicate skin cancer, but the risk of the mole turning malignant is definitely present. As for freckles, they are indirectly linked to the development of skin cancer. Unlike moles, freckles have no cellular structure. Instead, they are areas of the skin with a higher amount of pigment than others, and there is no risk of them becoming malignant. However, studies do show that children with a large number of freckles are at a higher risk for developing skin cancer.

Some studies have indicated that gender may be a contributing factor in melanoma cases. For instance, women develop melanoma more frequently than men. There is no biological explanation for this, but epidemiologists believe that women are diagnosed with melanoma more frequently because they spend more time sunbathing. Even though women seem more likely to develop melanoma than men, they have a higher survival rate. There is no biological explanation for this either, but epidemiologists have speculated that women may pay more attention to their bodies, and notice changes in moles at an early enough stage, before metastasis. Still, melanoma is the leading cause of cancer deaths in women between the ages of twenty-four and twenty-nine.

Other people at risk for developing melanoma are those with defective immune systems. They include people with AIDS, lymphomas, or people on immunosuppressive medication after undergoing an organ transplant.

ENVIRONMENTAL RISK FACTORS

The sun provides our planet with energy through the waves that it emits. Mild exposure to the sun can be beneficial. Its wavelengths can kick off a chemical and metabolic chain reaction in your body that produces vitamin D, which is proven to promote bone health. However, excessive exposure is harmful for the skin. The sun gives off three types of electromagnetic radiation that are relevant to skin cancer and melanoma: visible radiation is the light from the sun that we can see; infrared radiation is the warmth that we feel from the sun; ultraviolet radiation is invisible and is a carcinogen, meaning that it is capable of both initiating a malignancy and promoting its growth. UV radiation is the most harmful to your skin.

UV rays are divided into three groups, based on wavelengths and frequency: UVA, UVB, and UVC. UVA has the longest wavelength and lowest frequency, while UVC has the shortest wavelength and highest frequency. UVA radiation remains constant year-round, regardless of the season; is the type of radiation emitted from tanning booths;

EPIDEMIOLOGY

Epidemiology is a type of science that studies how often and why diseases occur in a population of people, as well as the distribution and progression of an illness. The information collected is used to plan strategies for prevention, treatment, and a cure. The epidemiology of melanoma is important because the number of diagnosed cases rises at an alarming rate each year. Until the number of cases lowers or at least stabilizes, it is clear that melanoma research is still very crucial.

and can cause sunburn. Because of its long wavelength, UVA rays can penetrate deep into the layers of the skin, accelerating the skin changes associated with aging, like wrinkles and loss of elasticity. UVA can cause damage to the DNA of skin cells, thus resulting in cancer. Research has shown that it is also an immunosuppressive agent. This means that it can significantly deplete the skin's immune cells, giving growth advantage to malignant cells, rendering UVA radiation as a tumor promoter.

UVB is the most damaging of the UV bands. As a tumor initiator, it causes all types of skin cancer, including melanoma. Like UVA, UVB radiation causes sunburn and accelerates the effects of aging, damages the DNA of skin cells, and is a tumor promoter. The intensity of UVB rays varies. UVB rays are more concentrated in the summer, at higher altitudes, at certain times of the day, and at latitudes that are close to the equator. Earth is a sphere, so landmasses closer to the equator are closer to the sun. For example, in the United States, UVB rays are much more intense in Florida than in Maine.

UVC has the potential to be the most harmful of the UV rays, but because of our ozone layer, most of the UVC rays are absorbed and never

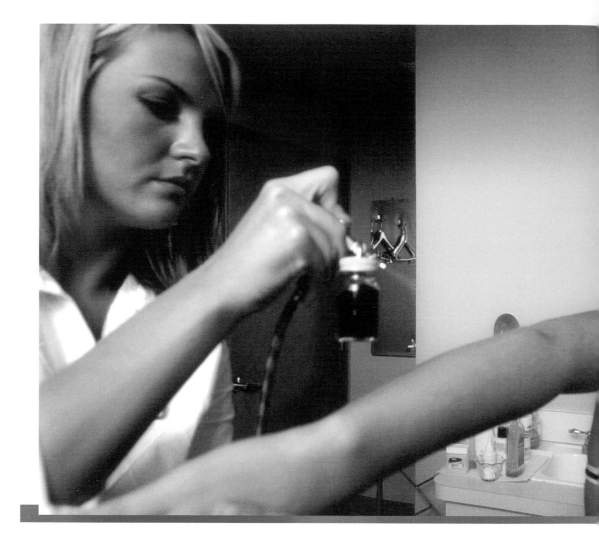

even reach Earth's surface. However, as the ozone layer depletes from pollution, more UVC rays are able to reach Earth's surface, increasing the risk of all forms of skin cancer. It is estimated that for each 10 percent decrease in the ozone layer, there will be a 30 percent increase in squamous cell cancer, 50 percent increase in basal cell cancer, and 10 percent increase in malignant melanoma.

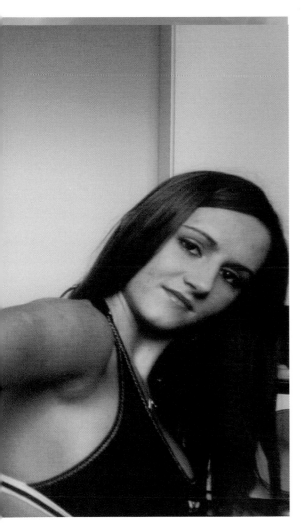

One safe alternative to tanning in the sun or on an indoor bed is the increasingly popular spray-on tan. Because tans from spray-on solutions and lotions are obtained by chemical reaction, they do not put the skin at the same risk as harmful UV rays.

Wind and reflections from surfaces like water, sand, and snow increase the damaging effects of UV rays. Even on cloudy days, it is estimated that 85 percent of the total UV radiation of the sun reaches Earth's surface. The melanin pigment in skin absorbs and detoxifies UV rays. Therefore, darker skin is more protected from UV rays than fair skin because it has more melanin.

Melanoma is most commonly associated with heavy, intermittent exposure to the sun. For example, a person who spends most of his or her time indoors, but exposes his or her skin to a large amount of sun on weekends and vacations is at great risk. But long-term exposure to the sun can be just as dangerous, affecting older people with sun-damaged skin. However, it may be the early exposure that matters most. According to a study published in the *Journal of the National Cancer Institute* in 2003, severe sunburns received when a person is under the age of twenty could cause the most damage to his or her skin later in life. Doctors also advise patients to avoid artificial tans from tanning booths. Tanning booths emit UVA rays, which can cause nonmelanoma skin cancer, and can work together with UVB rays to trigger melanoma. There is a misconception held by some people that getting a "base tan" in a tanning booth will help to protect skin from harmful UV rays outdoors. This is not true. The only truly safe way to tan is chemically, by using "bottled tans" to dye the top layers of the skin, which are made up of dead cells.

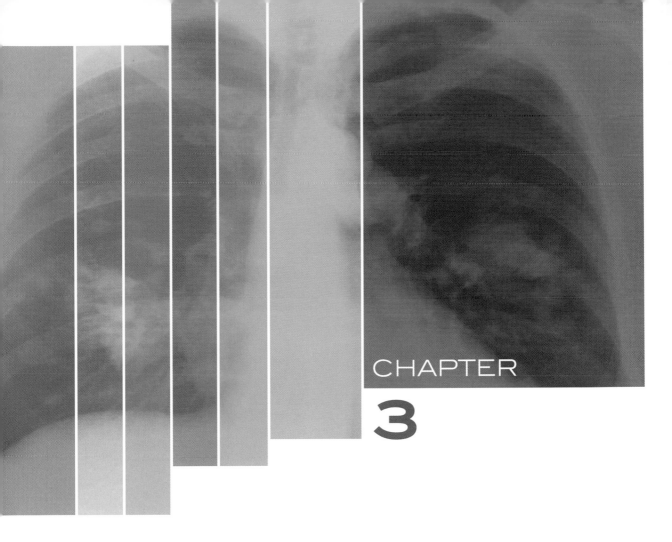

MELANOMA

When you think of melanoma, you probably think of cutaneous melanoma—melanoma that begins in the skin. However, melanoma can initiate in other parts of the body such as the eye, mouth, rectum, and vagina.

Cases of ocular melanoma are rare but serious. Ocular melanomas begin in the back of the eye, and the most common symptom is loss of vision in all or part of the eye. If they aren't diagnosed early enough, these melanomas commonly spread to the liver. The cause of ocular melanoma is unclear, as the back part of the eye isn't exposed to the

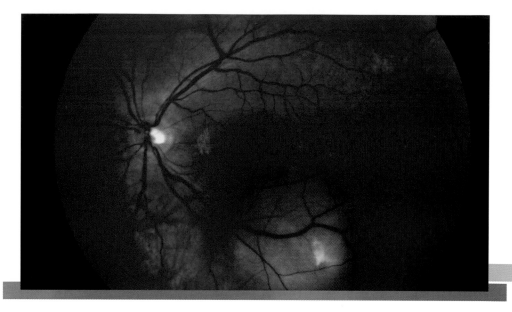

Though quite rare, ocular melanoma can be very dangerous. The image above shows choroidal malignant melanoma, the most common type of ocular melanoma. Located just behind the retina, the choroid is extremely pigmented, and once tainted by melanoma, its proximity to the optic nerve makes it likely that the melanoma will spread to other parts of the body.

sun. However, there is speculation that UV rays pass through the cornea and lens of the eye in childhood, triggering ocular melanoma later in life.

Mucosal melanoma occurs on the mucous membranes of the body: the mouth, rectum, and vagina. Another rare form, mucosal melanomas are not caused by sun exposure. Because it is difficult to diagnose, mucosal melanoma is frequently not discovered until it has spread to other parts of the body. The symptoms may vary, depending on where the melanoma starts, making this an obscure and particularly dangerous form of melanoma.

GROWTH PHASES

Melanomas do not start out malignant, thus they are not able to spread to the internal organs of the body until they have progressed through growth phases. Radial growth phase—during which the melanoma does not form a tumor, lump, or nodule—contains two steps. In the first step, the melanoma cells are contained entirely in the epidermis, and in the second step, the melanoma cells may slightly invade the dermis, but do not flourish there. If left untreated, the melanoma will move on to the next phase, the vertical growth phase. In this phase, the melanoma grows as a tumor in the dermis, creating a chance for the cancer to spread. To prevent a melanoma from becoming fatal, it is essential to remove it completely during its radial growth phase, before it moves on to the vertical growth phase.

CUTANEOUS MELANOMA

Cutaneous melanoma is broken down into subcategories, based on the appearance of the melanomas under the microscope.

The most common type is superficial spreading, which accounts for more than half of cutaneous melanoma cases. More frequent in women than men, they are typically found on the lower legs and back. Superficial spreading often develops from an existing mole, but can also initiate in an unblemished portion of skin. These lesions have irregular borders, are slightly raised, and are pigmented in variable shades of brown and black, but they can also have other colors, such as blue or red. Superficial, spreading lesions tend to grow laterally

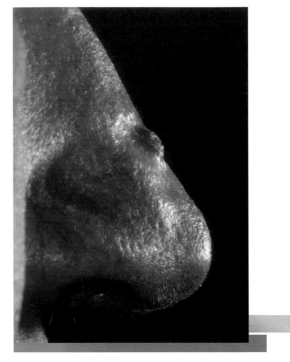

The growth on this man's nose is a basal cell carcinoma, which often occurs on parts of the body that are regularly exposed to sunlight. One potential danger regarding basal cell carcinomas is the fact that they look like other skin disorders such as psoriasis and eczema. It is important to have a physician examine these growths to make a proper diagnosis. Basal cell carcinomas can appear as open sores, red patches, white scar-like areas, shiny, pearly bumps, or pink growths.

along the skin for a long period of time before they begin to invade deeper. If the lesion is ignored, oozing, bleeding, or crusting can occur. The development of nodules or thickening is an indication that the tumor has entered the vertical, or invasive, growth phase, resulting in a rapidly worsening prognosis.

Nodular melanomas are most commonly found in men older than fifty, and make up 20 to 25 percent of cutaneous melanoma cases. Appearing, for the most part, on the head and neck, nodular lesions are dome-shaped, elevated above the level of the skin, and are dark brown or black. They tend to change in size, and may become associated with nearby smaller lesions, referred to as satellite lesions, indicating a local spread. Both nodular and superficial spreading melanomas are triggered by a combination of excessive sun exposure and skin sensitivity. Unlike superficial spreading, nodular lesions invade vertically very rapidly, resulting in a poorer prognosis than superficial spreading.

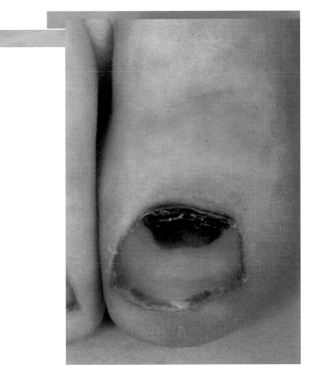

A toenail may seem like an unlikely site for a melanoma, but a dangerous malignancy can develop there. Because it is unexpected, this kind of melanoma is often misdiagnosed and the cancer isn't detected until it's too late. Acral lentiginous melanoma is the most common form of melanoma to affect dark skin. It begins as a flat black spot, usually on the palm or sole.

Lentigo maligna melanomas are less common than nodular and superficial spreading melanomas. They are mostly found in people older than the age of sixty who have long histories of heavy sun exposure. Usually found on the face, lentigo maligna melanomas can also appear on other sun-exposed areas such as hands and legs, and are not developed from moles. With lentigo maligna melanoma, there is a long, preinvasive phase that can go on for many years, during which the lesion appears as a flat, light brown stain on the skin. The development of an elevated nodule is an indication of vertical growth.

The types of melanoma already discussed in this chapter tend to occur in Caucasian skin. However, acral lentiginous melanoma, a rare form of the disease, occurs equally in light and dark skinned people, and does not appear to be caused by sun exposure. It appears most frequently on the palms of hands, soles of feet, undersurface of fingers and toes, and under nails. An acral lentiginous lesion appears as a large, flat,

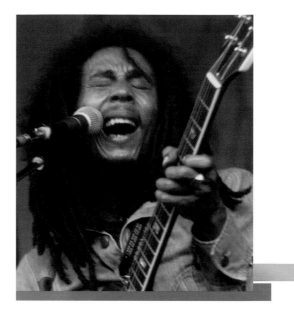

Music legend Bob Marley (right) assumed the wound under his toenail was the result of a soccer injury. When the wound wouldn't heal—and when the nail fell off—he consulted a doctor, who diagnosed it as a malignant melanoma. Marley refused recommendations to amputate the toe, arguing such a procedure went against his Rasta beliefs, and the cancer metastasized to his brain and lungs.

pigmented area that may bleed or ooze. Of the areas that can be affected by this type of melanoma, thumbnails and big toe nails are most common. When a lesion affects the nail, the melanoma begins at the base and creates a streak toward the tip of the nail. Tumors that start in the nail are often misdiagnosed, thought of as old blood from recent trauma to the nail. Acral lentiginous melanoma is the type of cancer that reggae music legend Bob Marley had. It began in his big toe, and eventually spread to his lungs and brain, resulting in his death in 1981.

Desmoplastic melanomas, or neurotrophic melanomas, and amelanotic melanomas are highly unusual, and because of their rarity, not much is known about them. Neither makes pigment, so lesions appear as pink or flesh colored. Due to the lack of pigment, these lesions are often misdiagnosed as pimples or other nonmalignant lesions.

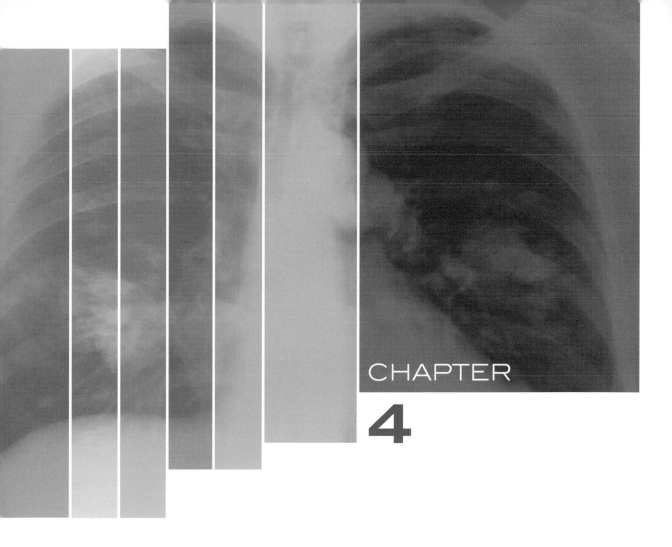

DETECTION AND DIAGNOSIS

Early detection is the best weapon in fighting skin cancer. Carefully watching suspicious moles is a good start. There are several things to look for in determining whether or not a mole should be further evaluated. The ABCDE checklist below has been developed by the American Cancer Society as an easy reference.

A stands for "asymmetry," which means disproportionate or unbalanced. When looking at a mole, look for signs of asymmetry, where one half of the lesion appears structurally different from the other, giving it an irregular shape.

B stands for "border." The borders of a mole should be a smooth oval or rounded shape. Border irregularities, such as notches, where it looks like "bites" have been taken out of the mole, are an indication of a melanoma.

C stands for "color." Normal moles have one color. Melanomas can be different hues of brown, black, blue, pink, red, or even white. Any variation in color is a warning sign.

D stands for "diameter" (the measurement from one point to another through the center of a circle). Because melanomas grow to be larger than regular moles, a pigmented area that is larger than six millimeters in diameter, or a mole that is clearly growing, may be a problem.

E stands for "elevation." Any pigmented lesion that becomes elevated or develops a bump should be checked out immediately.

Any other change in a lesion, such as itchiness or bleeding, should prompt a doctor's evaluation. The ABCDE checklist is a good way to initially identify whether a mole may be cancerous. However, the only real way to determine this is through a biopsy.

BIOPSIES

A person concerned about a changing mole should see a doctor and then, if necessary, a dermatologist. If the dermatologist is unable to determine whether or not the suspicious mole is cancerous, then a biopsy will be required. A biopsy is the surgical removal of tissue to be

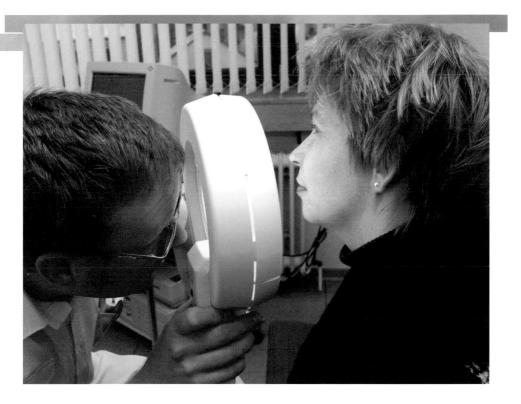

A dermatologist will closely examine a patient's skin, looking through special magnifiers for signs of damage. People with an abundance of moles should have their bodies "mapped" annually by their dermatologist. Mapping involves carefully studying the skin for moles and recording their size, appearance, and location. The dermatologist can consult the map to see if any of the moles have grown or changed considerably.

examined under a microscope in order to establish a precise diagnosis. Once a biopsy is done, it can take anywhere from two to seven days to get the diagnostic report back. A biopsy is a relatively simple procedure, usually conducted on an outpatient basis using a local anesthetic to numb the area. Different biopsy techniques are used, depending on the size and location of the tissue in question.

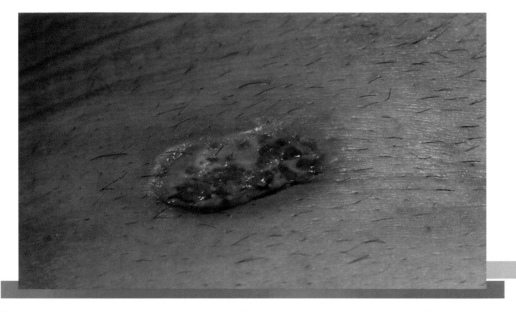

This photograph shows a squamous cell carcinoma that was removed in a punch biopsy. Punch biopsies are generally used to obtain a large or intact sample. The blade is pushed through the epidermis and dermis, and into the subcutaneous fat, and the specimen is removed and studied.

The easiest and most employed is the shave biopsy. In this biopsy technique, a lesion is elevated from the skin with a pair of forceps, and a scalpel is used to cut the lesion away. The downside to this simple procedure is that some of the lesion may be left behind. If this is the case, and the diagnostic report indicates melanoma, another procedure will have to be performed to remove the rest of the tissue.

A punch biopsy uses a tool called a punch scalpel, which looks like a small tube with a very sharp edge that comes in different diameters for different sized lesions. The punch scalpel is twisted, cutting into the skin, the way a cookie cutter cuts into dough. Scissors are used to cut the last portion of the connected tissue away.

MOHS SURGERY

When a suspected malignant lesion is removed, so is some of the normal tissue surrounding it, just to make sure that no malignant cells are left behind. In some cases, a skin graft is required. A skin graft is the process of removing a piece of skin from one part of the body and transferring it to an area where wound closure is difficult due to excessive skin removal. This process is not popular with patients because it leaves a scar. Mohs surgery, developed by Dr. Frederick Mohs in the 1930s, is a technique in which the tissue is immediately examined under the microscope to make sure the margins are clear. This surgery enables doctors to remove small pieces of tissue at a time, until they have removed the entire tumor, with little scarring. Mohs surgery takes several hours, and is typically only performed on areas such as the face, where scarring or disfiguring would be traumatic.

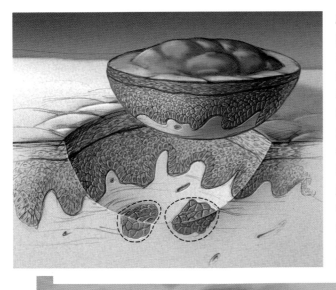

Mohs surgery removes any fear that the tissue surrounding a malignancy could still be affected. As shown in the illustration at left, the melanoma is completely excised, leaving no cancerous tissue or roots behind. Because Mohs surgery allows the greatest control in terms of removing lesions, recurrences are less likely than with other types of removal.

An incisional biopsy is performed on larger lesions appearing on parts of the body, such as the face, that may require specialized surgery. A scalpel is used to cut away a small portion of the tissue in question. Like shave and punch biopsies, disturbance to the skin's appearance is minimal with incisional biopsies.

Excisional biopsies are a little more invasive. Thought to be the best and most thorough, excisional biopsies remove the entire lesion, as well as some normal tissue around it with a scalpel and scissors. A few stitches are required to close the wound. Excisional biopsies often are performed when the lesion is highly suspicious of a malignancy.

CLASSIFICATION

If a lesion has been biopsied and diagnosed as a melanoma, there are two characteristics doctors consider when determining a prognosis and deciding on a treatment plan: the lesion's growth phase and its likelihood of metastasis. In 1969, Dr. Wallace Clark was the first to distinguish between melanomas that would not spread beyond their original site (radial growth phase) and melanomas that had the ability to spread beyond their original site (vertical growth phase). He also categorized melanomas in five different levels measuring the depth of tumor penetration into skin layers. This classification system would become known as Clark level.

Level I Lesions grow along the dermal/epidermal junction and are not metastatic, because they haven't invaded deep into the skin. They pose no fatal risk to the person diagnosed.

Level II Lesions have broken through the dermal/epidermal junction to partially invade the papillary layer. These lesions are the first level of invasion that may spread, but they tend to carry a low risk for metastasis.

Level III Lesions invade deeper into the skin, to the border of the papillary and reticular layers of the dermis, with a risk of metastatic spread.

Level IV Lesions invade straight through to the reticular layer, and although they do not reach the subcutaneous tissue, they are at high risk for metastasis.

Level V Lesions have invaded straight through to the subcutaneous tissue and carry the highest risk of all the levels for metastatic spread.

In the early 1970s, just a few years after Dr. Clark developed the Clark level, Dr. Alexander Breslow developed a different classification system—called Breslow thickness—for lesions that have penetrated below the epidermis, based on the thickness of the melanoma. A measurement device is now incorporated into the eyepieces of microscopes to enable pathologists to directly measure the thickness and depth of the melanoma. The stage of the melanoma is then classified according to the T staging system.

T0 A radial growth melanoma that hasn't invaded into the skin.

T1 A tumor that is up to one millimeter thick.

T2 A tumor that is more than one but no more than two millimeters thick.

T3 A tumor that is more than two but no more than four millimeters thick.

T4 A tumor that is more than four millimeters thick.

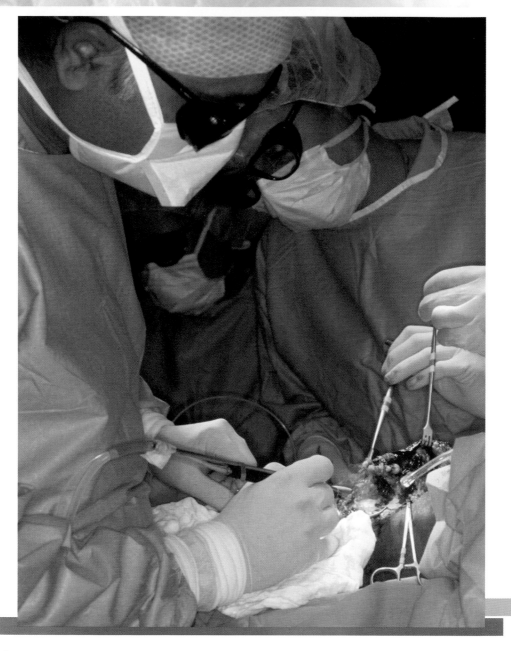

Some skin cancers must be removed surgically, as discussed in the next chapter.
Here, doctors use a YAG laser to remove a squamous cell carcinoma from a
patient's leg. Laser removal often must be performed in stages. The laser's high
heat leads to easy cell death.

Although Clark level and Breslow thickness are both given in a pathologist's report, many believe the latter to be of more use when planning further surgical treatment.

METASTASIS

As discussed earlier, metastasis is the process by which cancer spreads from its starting point to other areas of the body. Melanoma metastasizes when the tumor invades the skin in the vertical growth phase, in which the melanoma cells gain access to blood and lymphatic vessels, allowing the cells to travel to other parts of the body. When the malignant cells enter an organ, they begin to multiply, forming individual tumors, and eventually displace normal cells, interfering with the function of organs and compromising the health of the individual. Once the melanoma cells begin to spread this way, a chance for a cure significantly decreases.

The symptoms of metastatic melanoma vary depending on the site of the spread, but there are some general warning signs. For instance, unexplained fatigue; swelling in the skin; unexplained persistent pain; loss of appetite; and shortness of breath, though vague, can all be signals that a person has developed metastatic melanoma. The largest problem with metastatic disease in internal organs is that there may be too many tumors before symptoms become obvious.

Melanoma metastases fall into two general categories. Regional metastasis is confined to the region of the primary tumor, and encompasses nearby lymph nodes as well as the skin between those lymph nodes and the primary site. Regional metastases are usually surgically removed.

Distant metastases develop beyond the primary site and can spread to a number of organs in the body. Distant metastasis can occur in "nonregional" parts of the skin: lymph nodes, lungs, liver, bones, and the brain. Apart from the spreading to the skin, which is quite visible, most of these locations for metastasis go undetected, accounting for most of the fatalities attributed to malignant melanoma.

TREATMENT

Oncology is a field of medicine that focuses on the study and treatment of cancer. An oncologist is a doctor who specializes in the care of cancer patients. After a primary care physician or dermatologist has performed the surgical removal of a melanoma lesion, he or she may refer the patient to an oncologist, who will determine whether additional therapy is needed. If a melanoma lesion has not metastasized, then, most likely, an oncologist will not suggest additional therapy. However, if a melanoma lesion has metastasized, spreading to other parts of the body, additional therapy will most likely be necessary for any chance of survival. An oncologist will perform specialized tests such as PET (positron-emission tomography) and CAT (computerized axial tomography) scans to determine if and how much the cancer has spread. The oncologist will then work with the patient to determine the best treatment option, and usually will administer that treatment to the patient.

It's important for a patient to understand and accept his or her oncologist's treatment philosophy. For instance, some patients want to approach their treatment immediately and aggressively, and are willing to suffer any physical pain or sickness that side effects may bring, for even a small chance of a benefit. Other patients are more interested in their quality of life, and will only undergo harsh treatment if it has a very good chance for a successful outcome. Also, some doctors may believe only in a traditional path toward battling cancer, such as chemotherapy and immunotherapy. However, there are many patients who believe in the benefits of alternative therapies regarding diet and lifestyle.

SURGERY

The first decision an oncologist makes when determining treatment is whether to surgically remove the cancer. Factors such as location, the number of tumors, and medical problems of the patient are key in deciding if surgery will be beneficial. The most common side effect of surgery is pain on the site where the operation was performed, lasting from twenty-four to forty-eight hours, due to the disruption of the normal nerve pathways. Other side effects include cosmetic damage due to scarring, or infection of the area where the incision was made.

If the surgeon is able to remove all of the cancer cells, then the surgery is considered a success. However, with metastasized cancer, some

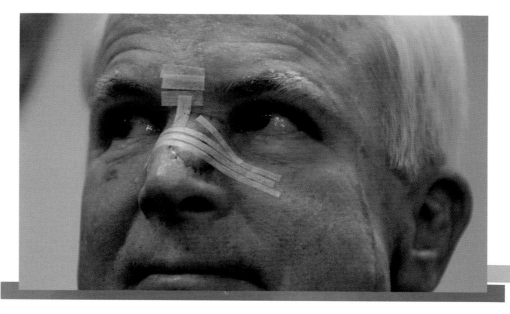

Senator John McCain (above) *made a public appearance in 2002 wearing bandages that covered scars from a recent procedure to remove a cancerous lesion. McCain visited a doctor at the first sign of trouble, and fortunately his melanoma was diagnosed and treated before it had metastasized.*

forms of which can spread rapidly, that is rarely the case. Since surgery can only remove visible elements of the disease, and will not treat microscopic elements, some form of adjuvant therapy is usually combined with this treatment. While surgery does not usually effect a cure from these secondary cancers, many physicians believe that it provides a degree of relief and an improved quality of life.

RADIATION

Radiation therapy involves the delivery of treatment for metastatic melanoma through a radioactive source. Like surgery, the radiation treats the visible parts of the disease, in addition to some surrounding normal tissue. Administered anywhere between one to six weeks at a

PET AND CAT SCANS

Positron-emission tomography (PET) and computerized axial tomography (CAT) scans are highly specialized tests that are able to find very small tumors that may have spread from the primary site. While a PET scan provides metabolic detail, a CAT scan provides anatomic detail. A PET scan is a test that uses a small amount of radioactive glucose instead of X-rays to identify areas of the body with tumor cells. A CAT scan is a specialized procedure that uses X-rays reproduced by a computer to take pictures of cross-sections of the body in order to look for tumors. CAT scans use more radiation than a chest X-ray, but the benefits of the procedure generally outweigh the harm. PET and CAT scans can be performed at the same time, with the procedure lasting about thirty minutes. In the majority of cases, if melanoma metastasizes, it will do so within two years after the patient's initial diagnosis. CAT and PET scans are performed every four months for those first two years, and eventually decrease over time, as the likelihood of recurrence declines.

time, radiation therapy treats an area by using a CAT scan, wherein the area to be treated is identified and mapped.

In many cases, metastatic lesions are found to be responsive to radiation. However, like surgery, radiation is not the most efficient way of catching an entire metastasis, and supplemental treatment is usually required. There are significant side effects to radiation, such as the inflammation of the skin in the irradiated area, similar to that of sunburn. Normal tissue surrounding a malignancy also can be damaged by the

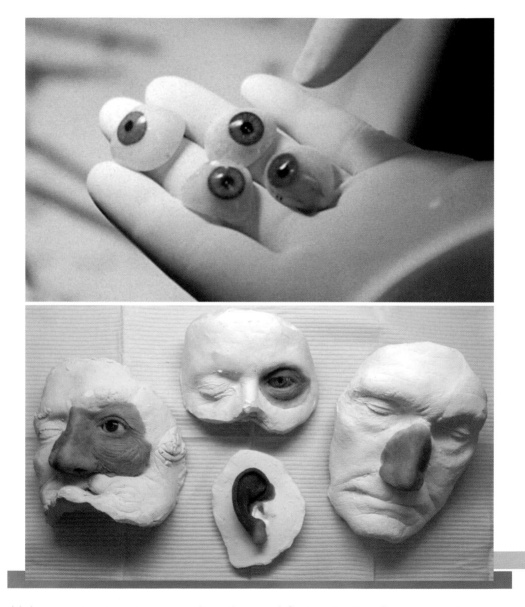

Melanoma treatment can result in the need for prosthetics. Since an ocular melanoma is often treated by complete removal of the eye, many patients opt for artificial replacements, as shown at top. Facial prosthetics made from plastics and silicone (bottom) can replace other parts of the face.

radiation. Radiation is typically used when surgery isn't appropriate, for instance, on the elderly, or patients who are not surgical candidates due to a physical condition.

IMMUNOTHERAPY, CHEMOTHERAPY, AND IMMUNOCHEMOTHERAPY

Under the right conditions, the body's immune system is capable of killing melanoma cells. The "right conditions" are not really known, despite intense research on the matter. However, an effective treatment known as immunotherapy has been developed to fight skin cancer. Immunotherapy is used as a local treatment to shrink secondary malignancies of the skin or the subcutaneous tissue.

An immune activating agent like Bacillus Calmette-Guérin (BCG) or interferon is injected directly into the tumor, which produces an inflammatory reaction that can wipe out melanoma. Immunologic agents do not kill the tumor directly, however. Instead, the agents stimulate the production of the body's immune cells, which recognize malignant cells as abnormal and then kill them. BCG and interferon are only two of several immunotherapy medications in use that all share similar side effects. Mostly, patients experience flulike symptoms such as fever, chills, muscle and joint pain, nausea, vomiting, and diarrhea. Immunotherapy isn't yet effective as a systemwide treatment of metastatic melanoma, however, it is very effective as a lesion-by-lesion treatment method.

When you think of cancer treatments, chemotherapy probably comes to mind, as it's the most common and well-known form of treatment for many different types of cancer. Chemotherapy (commonly referred to as chemo) treats cancer by using medication that directly kills malignant cells by disrupting their ability to divide and grow. Unfortunately, most chemotherapy agents not only attack malignant cells, but normal cells as well. Therefore, chemotherapy presents a

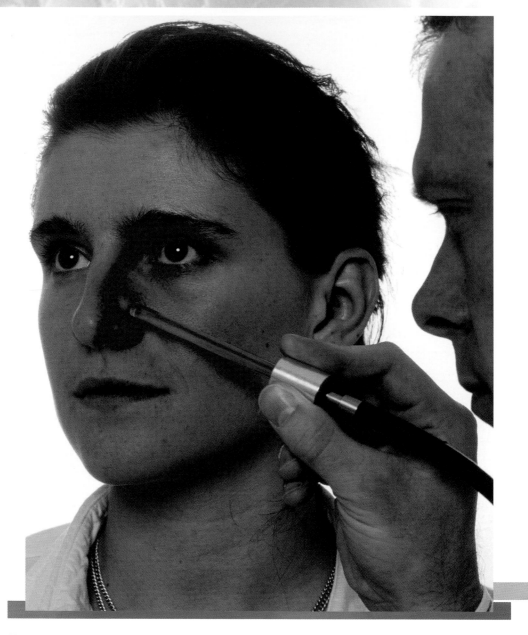

The Paterson PDT lamp, shown above, was invented in England and makes use of photodynamic therapy. It activates a reaction in a cream that is spread onto cancer cells, killing them without pain or scarring. The lamp is considered an improvement over lasers and is much cheaper, but it has been in use for less than ten years and is not as widely available.

number of adverse side effects, depending on which medication is used, such as the inability to eat, abdominal pain or bleeding, nausea, vomiting, and hair loss.

Advanced melanoma tends to be resistant to standard chemotherapy agents, so a combination of chemotherapy and immunotherapy, referred to as immunochemotherapy or biochemotherapy, is found to be more effective than using either of these methods on their own. According to a recent study conducted at Lutheran General Hospital in Chicago, the overall response to immunochemotherapy was extraordinarily high, at around 55 percent, with one in seven patients entering full remission.

Adjuvant therapy is any treatment given to supplement surgery when a disease is statistically likely to have metastasized, but no physical evidence of metastasis exists. Since adjuvant therapies are designed to kill microscopic parts of the disease that have spread to unknown areas, they generally affect the whole body. Until recently, there hadn't really been a successful adjuvant therapy for melanoma patients. However, with the development of interferon medication and continued clinical trials, there is hope for survival.

CLINICAL TRIALS

Clinical trials are tests on new drugs or drug combinations that are not yet approved by the Food and Drug Administration (FDA), or treatments to determine their effectiveness in fighting malignancies. Because there is no standard or completely effective treatment for metastatic melanoma, researching and testing new therapies is essential in developing a cure. Clinical trials have been extremely successful in developing treatments for breast cancer and other cancers. Participation in clinical trials is completely voluntary, and a patient must meet certain criteria in order to take part in a particular trial. Generally, patients must be at least eighteen years old, and their disease cannot be so advanced upon entering the trial that they are too ill to participate.

Clinical trials are designed to test treatments on certain situations or types of cancer. A protocol must be written, describing the rationale behind the trial, how treatment will be given, and who is eligible. The protocol is then submitted to the Institutional Review Board (IRB), where it is evaluated for scientific design and safety measures. Once a trial is approved by the IRB, it may begin. Information on the clinical trials being conducted is available from the National Cancer Institute.

There are three types of clinical trials: phases I, II, and III. Phase I trials are conducted to determine the correct dosage of a certain drug and how the body metabolizes it. Typically, only twenty to eighty people are required for this testing phase. If the trial is successful in phase I, it moves on to phase II, which tests the effectiveness of the drug for specific uses and the activity of the drug when used alone. Several hundred volunteers can participate in this phase. Phase III trials are conducted to determine the effectiveness of a new treatment in comparison to more standard treatments. Depending on the study, several hundred to several thousand may be enrolled. In a phase III trial, one set of patients receives the new treatment while another set receives a standard treatment. In order for the research to be unbiased, the patients are chosen at random and do not know which treatment they are being given. If there is no standard treatment for this particular form of cancer, one test group will be given placebos. The goal of phase III is to compare the benefits and hazards of the investigational treatment to the standard treatment.

Clinical trials are funded in different ways, depending on the sponsor. Sponsors may include pharmaceutical companies, cooperative groups of physicians, or the National Cancer Institute. Generally, patients do not pay for clinical trials.

There are definitely risks for a patient enrolled in a clinical trial, depending on what phase the testing is in. Phase I poses the most risk to the patient. Since it involves testing drugs never used before on humans, a patient is liable to develop toxic side effects. Since the correct doses are better known by phase II, there aren't as many unknown risks in phases II and III. However, in phase III, a test group receiving placebos receives no treatment or protection from their cancer at all.

ALTERNATIVE MEDICINE

Because there are very few effective treatments for metastatic melanoma, patients often look to alternative treatments. One alternative is the holistic approach to medicine. The philosophy behind holistic medicine is that it treats the patient as a whole person—body, mind, and spirit—rather than as a collection of symptoms. For the most part, holistic medicine combines traditional treatment with natural treatments like herbs, special diets, and homeopathy. Most alternative treatments, like herbal remedies and diets, are unproven as effective in fighting melanoma, so a patient should carefully evaluate the pros and cons before beginning any treatment.

CHAPTER

6

PREVENTION, SCREENINGS, AND THE IMPORTANCE OF FUNDING AND RESEARCH

Prevention of skin cancer is the ultimate goal of doctors and researchers, and that begins with educating the public. If people know how to determine their skin type and assess their risks, they can begin to decide which prevention methods will work best. Limiting exposure to the sun is a good step, but its necessity is reduced if properly applied sunscreen is worn. Sunscreen is made up of chemicals that are able to absorb UV rays before they can enter the skin and interact with a person's DNA.

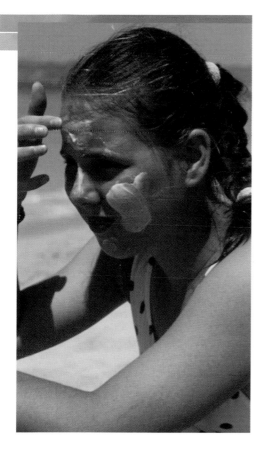

The good news about skin cancer is that most skin cancers are preventable. All you have to do is limit the contact your skin has with the sun. One way to prevent UV rays harming your skin is by applying sunscreen or sunblock. In fact, according to www.bioedonline.org, scientists are working on a sunscreen containing DNA fragments that can trick a wearer's own DNA into thinking it has damaged cells. This causes the reparation and manufacturing of new cells to kick into overdrive.

Sunblock is different in that it reflects rather than absorbs UV radiation energy. Either product is useful in the prevention of skin cancer. Many experts believe that wearing sunscreen or sunblock should be required for children the same way that wearing seat belts in cars is.

The term "SPF," found on sunscreen bottles, means "sun protection factor." The SPF number indicates how much protection is provided. One way to decide on which number SPF to use is to determine a person's minimal erythema dose (MED). MED is the measurement of how much time a person is able to stay in the sun before developing a light pink color. Multiplying those minutes by the SPF will determine how much time a person wearing that sunscreen can spend in the sun before turning light pink. So if a person turns pink after 15 minutes in the sun, he or she will be able to stay in the sun for 150 minutes

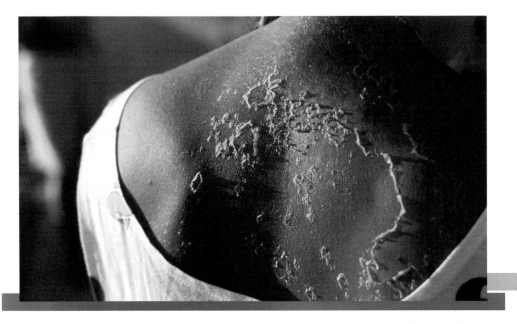

Extreme sunburns may result in swelling, blistering, or peeling, as shown above. Peeling is a reaction to the damage done to cells by the sun. Once damaged by UV rays, those cells are in danger of becoming cancerous. To protect itself, the body sheds them and allows new layers of cells to be generated.

wearing a sunscreen with an SPF of 10, before getting a light burn. If you want to spent two and a half hours in the sun, anything under SPF 10 won't do much to protect you from UV rays, and anything over SPF 20 won't provide much added protection, so anything between SPF 10 and SPF 20 is adequate.

There is a common misconception that sunscreen is not needed on cloudy days. However, UV rays are still strong on cloudy days and can still cause skin damage. Understanding the UV index is a good way to determine on which days it is necessary to wear sunscreen. The UV index was developed by the National Weather Service and the Environmental Protection Agency as a way to gauge how many minutes people should be exposed to the sun, unprotected, based on a scale of

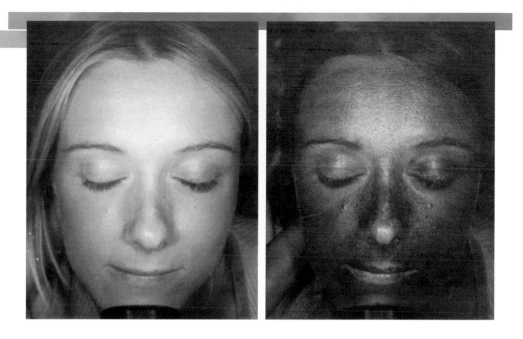

These photographs were taken with a special ultraviolet flash. What appears to be healthy skin on the left is actually quite damaged, as shown by the white patches in the photo on the right. Even normal daily exposure to the sun can lead to skin cancer, which is why dermatologists advise wearing some form of protection every day.

one to ten, ten being the most dangerous. The UV index is published every day in most newspapers.

SCREENINGS

Performing regular self-examinations using the ABCDE method to look for new and suspicious moles is an important component in the prevention of metastasis, because it enables melanoma moles to be caught at their earliest stage. Doctors suggest using a full-length mirror and a hand-held mirror, as well as a flashlight, to check every inch of the body. Professional skin examinations are also important. Mole checks are not an automatic procedure for most physicians, so they must be requested.

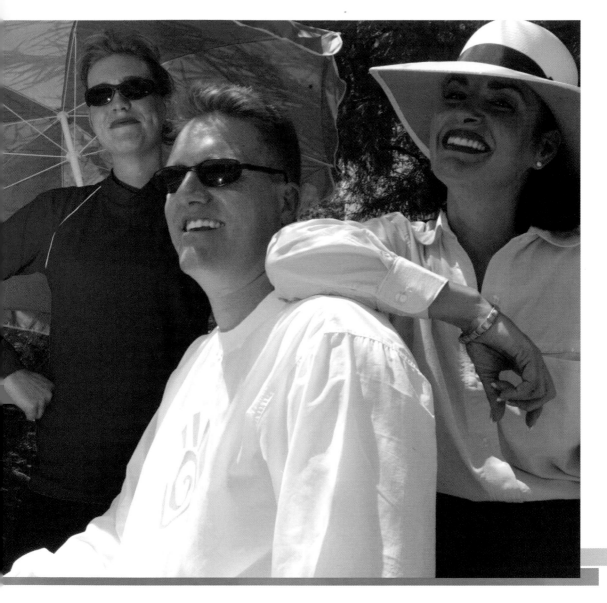

Manufacturers have created special protective clothing that has a tighter weave than normal fabrics and is designed to absorb UV rays before they can get to your skin. If you're going to be exposed to UV rays without wearing a sunscreen, it is important to wear a hat or carry an umbrella and to keep all skin covered.

ORGANIZATIONS FOR FUNDING, RESEARCH, AND AWARENESS

The American Academy of Dermatology (AAD) is a nonprofit organization dedicated to the promotion and advancement of research, medication, education, and patient care. Since 1985, the AAD has operated free screening programs for individuals without health care who are concerned that they may have a melanoma lesion. The National Cancer Institute and the American Mclanoma Foundation are also nonprofit organizations dedicated to educating the public, and raising funding for research. Because there aren't many truly effective ways to fight melanoma once it has metastasized, researching new methods is extremely important for saving the lives of those affected.

As with most types of cancer, the survival rate depends on how advanced the disease is when it is caught. For instance, nine of ten people who are diagnosed with melanoma in its first stage will be alive five years later. Naturally, survival rates decrease the later the stage of the disease when it is diagnosed. Only 20 percent to 30 percent of people who are diagnosed with melanoma in the final stage are likely to be alive five years later. And while there are new treatments being developed, and clinical trials being conducted, most doctors stress that the best weapon is early detection.

GLOSSARY

biopsy The removal and examination of a tissue sample from the body.

carcinogen A substance that is capable of causing cancer.

chemotherapy The treatment or control of cancer using anti-cancer drugs that destroy cancer cells by interfering with their growth or reproduction.

congenital Relating to a condition that is present at birth.

cutaneous Something relating to or affecting the skin.

dermatologist A doctor who specializes in the study and treatment of the skin.

dermis The layer of the skin that lies below the epidermis made up of connective tissue; it contains blood vessels, nerves, and glands.

diagnosis Identification of a disease in a person, made by a physician.

DNA (deoxyribonucleic acid) The material inside the nucleus of cells that carries genetic information.

dysplastic An abnormal development or growth of tissues, organs, and cells.

enzymes Proteins produced by the body to increase the speed of chemical reactions.

epidermis The outer layer of the skin.

homeopathy A system of treatment that uses the principle "like cures like." Small doses of medicines made from animals, plants, and minerals that would cause symptoms of the disease in a healthy person are given to a person suffering from that disease.

immunology A treatment that involves stimulating the body's own immune system to fight a disease.

immunosuppression Suppression of the immune system, either by drugs or radiation.

lesion A localized patch of skin that is diseased or infected.

malignant Tending to spread, deteriorate, and destroy.

melanocyte A skin cell that produces melanin and can be found in the basal layer of the epidermis.

metabolism All of the chemical processes that occur within a living cell.

metastasize To spread from one part of the body to another.

mutation The act or process of changing or being changed; a change of the DNA sequence within a gene or chromosome of an organism.

nodule A small mass of tissues that protrudes or bulges.

ocular Relating to the eye.

oncology The study of tumors.

ozone layer Layer about thirty miles (forty-eight kilometers) above Earth's surface that absorbs most of the sun's ultraviolet radiation.

pathologist A scientist who studies the nature of diseases as well as their causes, processes, development, and consequences.

pigment Natural coloring of plants and animals.

placebo A harmless substance that is often used in control experi-
ments to test the effectiveness of another medication.

prognosis A prediction, given by a doctor, of the course and outcome
of a disease.

radiation The emission of energy in the form of waves or rays.

remission The period after treatment when a cancer survivor is
cancer-free.

ulcer A lesion of the skin and mucous membrane.

FOR MORE INFORMATION

American Academy of Dermatology (AAD)
1350 I Street NW, Suite 880
Washington, DC 20005
(202) 842-3555
Web site: http://www.aad.org

American Cancer Society (ACS) National Home Office
1599 Clifton Road
Atlanta, GA 30329
(800) ACS-2345 (227-2345)
Web site: http://www.cancer.org

American Melanoma Foundation (AMF)
2160 Fletcher Pkwy, Suite O
El Cajon, CA 92020
(619) 448-0991
Web site: http://www.melanomafoundation.org

National Cancer Institute (NCI)
Cancer Information Service/CancerNet
Office of Cancer Communications
31 Center Drive
Building 31, Room 10A07
Bethesda, MD 20892
(800) 4-Cancer (422-6237)
Web site: http://www.nci.nih.gov

WEB SITES

Due to the changing nature of Internet links, the Rosen Publishing Group, Inc., has developed an online list of Web sites related to the subject of this book. This site is updated regularly. Please use this link to access the list:

http://www.rosenlinks.com/cms/skca

FOR FURTHER READING

Buchan, John, and Dafydd Lloyd Roberts. *Pocket Guide to Malignant Melanoma*. London, UK: Blackwell Science, 2000.

Kenet, Barney J., and Patricia Lawler. *Saving Your Skin: Prevention, Early Detection, and Treatment of Melanoma and Other Skin Cancers*. Emeryville, CA: Four Walls Eight Windows, 1998.

Long, Wendy. *Coping with Melanoma and Other Skin Cancers*. New York, NY: Rosen Publishing Group, 1999.

MacKie, Rona. *Primary and Secondary Prevention of Malignant Melanoma*. Switzerland: Karger, 1996.

McClay, Edward F., Mary T. McClay, and Jodie Smith. *100 Questions and Answers About Melanoma and Other Skin Cancers*. Sudbury, MA: Jones and Bartlett, 2004.

McNally, Robert Aquinas. *Skin Health Information for Teens: Health Tips About Dermatological Concerns and Skin Cancer Risks*. Detroit, MI: Omnigraphics, 2003.

Poole, Catherine M. with DuPont Guerry IV, MD. *Melanoma: Prevention, Detection, and Treatment*. New Haven, CT: Yale University Press, 1998.

Schofield, Jill R., and William A. Robinson. *What You Really Need to Know About Moles and Melanoma*. Baltimore, MD: Johns Hopkins University Press, 2000.

Spickler, Anna Rovid, *et al. Cancer Therapies: Awesome New Advances*. Angleton, TX: Biotech Publishing, 1998.

BIBLIOGRAPHY

Buchan, John, and Dafydd Lloyd Roberts. *Pocket Guide to Malignant Melanoma*. London, UK: Blackwell Science, 2000.

Eedy, D. J. "Surgical Treatment of Melanoma." *British Journal of Dermatology*, Vol. 149, No. 1, July 2003, pp. 2–12.

McClay, Edward F., Mary T. McClay, and Jodie Smith. *100 Questions and Answers About Melanoma and Other Skin Cancers*. Sudbury, MA: Jones and Bartlett, 2004.

Poole, Catherine M. *Melanoma: Prevention, Detection, and Treatment*. New Haven, CT: Yale University Press, 1998.

Spence, R. A. J., and P. G. Johnston, eds. *Oncology*. New York, NY: Oxford University Press, 2001.

Spickler, Anna Rovid. *Cancer Therapies: Awesome New Advances*. Angleton, TX: Biotech Publishing, 1998.

Teeley, Peter, and Philip Bashe. *The Complete Cancer Survival Guide*. New York, NY: Doubleday, 2000.

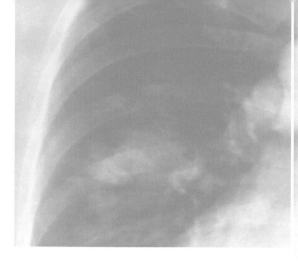

INDEX

ABOUT THE AUTHOR

Tracie Egan works for a women's magazine in New York City and has written many books for the Rosen Publishing Group. As someone who worries about excess exposure to the sun, Egan was interested to learn more about skin cancer and its prevention in researching this book.

PHOTO CREDITS

Cover © SPL/Photo Researchers; cover corner photo © PunchStock; back cover and throughout © National Cancer Institute; p. 5 © Bob Krist/Corbis; pp. 9, 11, 24, 26, 27, 32, 33, 36 © Custom Medical Medical Stock Photo; p. 12 © National Cancer Institute; pp. 15, 51 © Getty Images; p. 17 (right) Rafael Roa/Corbis, (left) Ann Brown/Superstock; pp. 20–21 © Anne Ryan/AP/Wide World Photos; p. 28 © Jeff Albertson/Corbis; p. 31 © Klaus Rose/Peter Arnold, Inc.; p. 40 © Stephen J. Boitano/AP/Wide World Photos; p. 42 © (top) Greg Fry/San Gabriel Valley Weekly/AP/Wide World Photos, (bottom) David Stephenson/Lexington Herald-Leader/AP/Wide World Photos; p. 44 © David Parker/Photo Researchers, Inc.; p. 49 © CC Studio/ Photo Researchers, Inc.; p. 50 © Peter Skinner/Photo Researchers, Inc.; p. 52 © Jennifer Grimes/East Valley Tribune/AP/Wide World Photos.

Designer: Evelyn Horovicz; Editor: Christine Poolos